MW01230727

The Vibrant Thai and Asian Meat Cookbook

The Complete Guide with 50 delicious Thai and Asian daily recipes

Madeline Soto

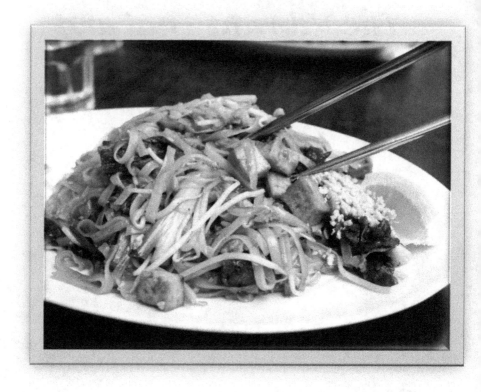

sources. Please consult a licensed professional before attempting any techniques outlined in this book.

By reading this document, the reader agrees that under no circumstances is the author responsible for any losses, direct or indirect, which are incurred as a result of the use of information contained within this document, including, but not limited to, — errors, omissions, or inaccuracies.

Table of contents

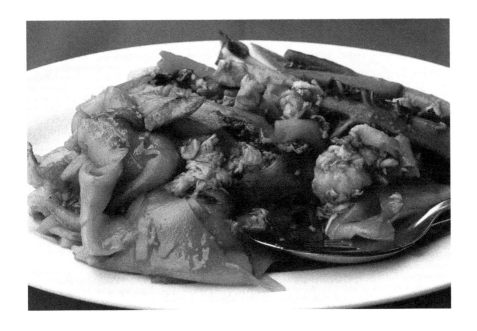

GREEN CURRY BEEF

Ingredients:

¼ cup (or to taste) Green Curry Paste

¼ cup brown sugar

¼ cup fish sauce

1 cup basil

1 pound eggplant (Japanese, Thai, or a combination), cut into ¼-inch slices

1½ pounds sirloin, cut into fine strips

2 cans coconut milk, thick cream separated from the milk

6 serrano chilies, stemmed, seeded, and cut in half along the length

Directions:

1. Put the thick cream from the coconut milk and the curry paste in a big soup pot and stir until blended. Put on moderate to high heat and bring to its boiling point. Decrease the heat and simmer for two to three minutes.

2. Put in the beef and the coconut milk, stirring to blend. Return the mixture to a simmer.

3. Put in the sugar and the fish sauce, stirring until the sugar dissolves, approximately 2 minutes.

4. Put in the eggplant and simmer for one to two minutes.

5. Put in the serrano chilies and cook one minute more.

6. Turn off the heat and mix in the basil.

Yield: Servings 4–6

CURRIED BEEF AND POTATO STEW

Ingredients:

¼ cup <u>Tamarind Concentrate</u>

½ cup brown sugar

½ cup unsalted roasted peanuts, chopped

½–¾ cup prepared Massaman Curry Paste

1 big onion, chopped

1 big russet potato, peeled and slice into bite-sized cubes

1 cup chopped fresh pineapple

1½ pounds beef stew meat, cut into bite-sized cubes 2 (14-ounce) cans coconut milk 2–3 tablespoons vegetable oil

7 tablespoons fish sauce

Jasmine rice, cooked in accordance with package directions

Directions:

1. Heat the oil in a big soup pot on moderate to high heat. Once the oil is hot, brown the meat on all sides. Put in the onion and cook until translucent, approximately two to three minutes.

2. Put in enough water to just cover the meat and onions. Bring to its boiling point, reduce heat, cover, and simmer for thirty to 60 minutes.

3. Put in the potatoes and carry on simmering for fifteen more minutes. (The potatoes will not be fairly thoroughly cooked now.)

4. Strain the solids from the broth, saving for later both.

5. In another soup pot, mix the coconut milk with the curry paste until well mixed. Bring the contents to a simmer on moderate to high heat and cook for two to three minutes.

6. Put in the reserved meat and potato mixture, the sugar, fish sauce, and tamarind, stirring until the sugar dissolves. Put in some of the reserved broth to thin the sauce to desired consistency.

7. Mix in the pineapple and carry on simmering until the potatoes are thoroughly cooked.

8. To serve, place some Jasmine rice in the center of individual serving plates and spoon the stew over the top. Decorate using the chopped peanuts.

Yield: Servings 4

RED BEEF CURRY

Ingredients:

¼ cup chopped basil

½ cup plus 2 tablespoons coconut milk

1 green or red sweet pepper, seeded and cubed

1 pound lean beef, cut into fine strips

1 tablespoon vegetable oil

1–3 tablespoons (to taste) fish sauce

2 tablespoons (roughly) ground peanuts

2 tablespoons <u>Red Curry Paste</u>

Rice, cooked in accordance with package directions Sugar to taste

Directions:

1. Heat the oil in a big sauté pan using low heat. Put in the curry paste and cook, stirring continuously, until aromatic, approximately one minute.

2. Mix in the ½ cup of coconut milk and bring the mixture to a simmer. Put in the beef strips and poach for five minutes.

3. Put in the peanuts and continue to poach for another five minutes.

4. Put in the fish sauce and sugar to taste; carry on cooking until the mixture is almost dry, then put in the sweet pepper and basil and cook for 5 more minutes.

5. Serve with rice.

Yield: Servings 4

HOT AND SOUR BEEF

Ingredients:

1 green onion, trimmed and thinly cut

1 tablespoon dark, sweet soy sauce

1 tablespoon fish sauce

1 tablespoon lime juice

1 teaspoon chopped cilantro

1 teaspoon dried chili powder

1 teaspoon honey

1½ pound sirloin steak

3 tablespoons chopped onion

Salt and pepper to taste

Directions:

1. Make the sauce by meticulously combining the first 8 ingredients; set aside.

2. Flavour the steak with salt and pepper, then grill or broil it to your preferred doneness. Take away the steak from the grill, cover using foil, and allow to rest for five to ten minutes.
3. Thinly slice the steak, cutting across the grain.

4. Position the pieces on a serving platter or on 1 or 2 dinner plates. Ladle the sauce over the top. Serve with rice and a side vegetable.

Yield: Servings 1–2

GRILLED GINGER BEEF

Ingredients:

1 (2-inch) piece of ginger, minced

1 (3-inch) piece ginger, cut in half

1 cinnamon stick

1 onion, cut in half

1 pound green vegetables

1 small package of rice noodles

2 dried red chili peppers

2 stalks lemongrass

2 tablespoons (or to taste) soy sauce

5 cloves garlic

6 (6-ounce) strip steaks

6 scallions, minced

8 cups low-salt beef broth

Salt and pepper to taste

Directions:

16

1. Put the beef broth, lemongrass, and garlic in a big pot; bring to its boiling point.

2. Meanwhile, put the ginger and onion halves, cut-side down, in a dry frying pan using high heat and cook until black. Put in the onion and ginger to the broth mixture.

3. Put the cinnamon and dried chili peppers in the dry frying pan and toast on moderate heat for a minute; put in to the broth mixture.

4. Lower the heat and simmer the broth for a couple of hours. Cool, strain, and place in your fridge overnight.

5. Before you are ready to eat, remove the broth from the fridge and skim off any fat that may have collected. Bring the broth to a simmer and put in the minced ginger.

6. Soak the rice noodles in hot water for ten to twenty minutes or until soft; drain.

7. Blanch the vegetables for approximately one minute. Using a slotted spoon, remove them from the boiling water and shock them in cold water.

8. Flavour the broth to taste with the soy sauce. Flavour the steaks

with salt and pepper and grill or broil to your preference.

9. To serve, slice the steaks into fine strips (cutting across the grain) and put them in 6 big bowls. Put in a portion of noodles and vegetables to the bowls and ladle the broth over the top.

Yield: Servings 6

THAI BEEF WITH RICE NOODLES

Ingredients:

¼ cup soy sauce

½ pound dried rice noodles

¾ pound sirloin, trimmed of all fat, washed and patted dry

1 pound greens (such as spinach or bok choy), cleaned and slice into ½-inch strips

2 eggs, beaten

2 tablespoons dark brown sugar

2 tablespoons fish sauce

2 tablespoons minced garlic

5 tablespoons vegetable oil, divided Crushed dried red pepper flakes to taste Freshly ground black pepper Rice vinegar to taste

Directions:

1. Cut the meat into two-inch-long, ½–inch-wide strips.

2. Cover the noodles with warm water for five minutes, then drain.

3. In a small container, mix the soy sauce, fish sauce, brown sugar, and black pepper; set aside.

4. Heat a wok or heavy frying pan using high heat. Put in roughly 2 tablespoons of the vegetable oil. Once the oil is hot, but not smoking, put in the garlic. After stirring for 5 seconds, put in the greens and stir-fry for roughly two minutes; set aside.

5. Put in 2 more tablespoons of oil to the wok. Put in the beef and

 stir-fry until browned on all sides, approximately 2 minutes; set aside.

6. Heat 1 tablespoon of oil in the wok and put in the noodles. Toss until warmed through, roughly two minutes; set aside.

7. Heat the oil remaining in the wok. Put in the eggs and cook, without stirring until they are set, approximately half a minute. Break up the eggs slightly and mix in the reserved noodles, beef, and greens, and the red pepper flakes. Mix the reserved soy mixture, then put in it to the wok. Toss to coat and heat through. Serve instantly with rice vinegar to drizzle over the top.

Yield: Servings 2–4

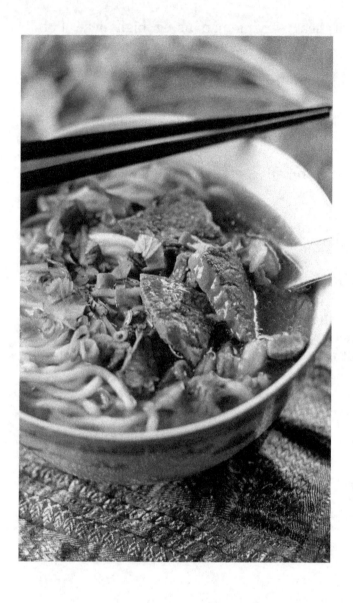

MINTY STIR-FRIED BEEF

Ingredients:

¼ cup chopped garlic

¼ cup chopped yellow or white onion

¼ cup vegetable oil

½ cup chopped mint leaves

½–¾ cup water

1 pound flank steak, cut across the grain into fine strips

1 tablespoon sugar

3 tablespoons fish sauce

7–14 (to taste) serrano chilies, seeded and crudely chopped

Directions:

1. Using a mortar and pestle or a food processor, grind together the chilies, garlic, and onion.

2. Heat the oil on moderate to high heat in a wok or big frying pan. Put in the ground chili mixture to the oil and stir-fry for one to two minutes.

3. Put in the beef and stir-fry until it just starts to brown.

4. Put in the rest of the ingredients, adjusting the amount of water

 depending on how thick you desire the sauce.

5. Serve with sufficient Jasmine rice.

Yield: Servings 4–6

CHILIED BEEF

Ingredients:

¼ cup white vinegar

1 big red onion, cut

1 pound flank steak

1 teaspoon dried red pepper flakes

2 tablespoons fish sauce

3 serrano chilies, stems removed and cut

4 scallions, trimmed and thinly cut

Bibb or romaine lettuce leaves

Juice of 1 big lime

Directions:

1. Put the cut chilies in a small container with the vinegar; allow it to stand for minimum fifteen minutes.

2. Grill or broil the flank steak to your desired doneness. Remove from the grill, cover using foil, and allow it to stand ten minutes. Thinly slice the streak across the grain.

3. Put the beef slices in a big container. Put in the red onion, scallions, lime juice, and red pepper flakes; toss all of the ingredients together. Cover the dish, place in your fridge, and let marinate for minimum 1 hour.

4. Before you serve, let the beef return to room temperature. Mound the beef on top of lettuce leaves and serve with white rice. Pass the serrano/vinegar sauce separately.

Yield: Servings 4–6

PORK AND EGGPLANT STIR-FRY

Ingredients:

3 tablespoons vegetable oil

½ pound ground pork

½ teaspoon freshly ground pepper

1 tablespoon fish sauce

1 tablespoon <u>Yellow Bean Sauce</u>

1 pound Japanese eggplant, cut into ¼-inch slices ¼ cup chicken stock

2 tablespoons (or to taste) sugar

5–10 cloves garlic, mashed

Directions:

1. Heat the oil in a wok or big frying pan on moderate to high heat. Once the oil is hot, put in the garlic and stir-fry until aromatic, approximately half a minute.

2. Put in the pork and continue to stir-fry until the pork loses its color, approximately one minute.

3. Put in the pepper, fish sauce, bean sauce, and eggplant; cook for a minute.

4. Put in the chicken stock. Continue to stir-fry for a couple of minutes.

5. Mix in the sugar to taste and cook until the eggplant is thoroughly cooked, approximately 2 more minutes.

Yield: Servings 2–4

PORK WITH GARLIC AND CRUSHED BLACK PEPPER

Ingredients:

4 tablespoons vegetable oil

1 pork tenderloin, trimmed of all fat and slice into medallions about ¼-inch thick

¼ cup sweet black soy sauce

2 tablespoons brown sugar

2 tablespoons fish sauce

2–2½ teaspoons black peppercorns, crudely ground 10–20 garlic cloves, mashed

Directions:

1. Put the garlic and the black pepper in a small food processor and process for a short period of time to make a crude paste; set aside.

2. Heat the oil in a wok or big frying pan on moderate to high heat. Once the oil is hot, put in the garlic-pepper paste and stir-fry until the garlic turns gold.

3. Increase the heat to high and put in the pork medallions; stir-fry for half a minute.

4. Put in the soy sauce and brown sugar, stirring until the sugar is dissolved.

5. Put in the fish sauce and carry on cooking until the pork is thoroughly cooked, approximately another one to two minutes.

Yield: Servings 2

BANGKOK-STYLE ROASTED PORK TENDERLOIN

Ingredients:

¼ teaspoon ground cardamom

¼ teaspoon ground ginger

¼–½ teaspoon freshly ground black pepper

½ cup chicken, pork, or vegetable stock, or water

1 teaspoon salt

2 (1-pound) pork tenderloins, trimmed Olive oil

Directions:

1. Put rack on bottom third of the oven, then preheat your oven to 500 degrees.

2. Mix the spices in a small container.

3. Rub each of the tenderloins with half of the spice mixture and a small amount of olive oil. Put the tenderloins in a roasting pan and cook for about ten minutes.

4. Turn the tenderloins over and roast for ten more minutes or until done to your preference.

5. Move the pork to a serving platter, cover using foil, and allow to rest.

6. Pour off any fat that has collected in the roasting pan. Put the pan on the stovetop using high heat and put in the stock (or water). Bring to its boiling point, scraping the bottom of the pan to loosen any cookedon bits. Sprinkle with salt and pepper to taste.

7. To serve, slice the tenderloins into thin slices. Pour a small amount of the sauce on top, passing more separately at the table.

Yield: Servings 4

CHIANG MAI BEEF

Ingredients:

1 pound lean ground beef

1 tablespoon chopped garlic

1 tablespoon small dried chilies

1 tablespoon vegetable oil

2 cups uncooked long-grained rice

2 green onions, trimmed and cut

3¼ cups water

3–4 tablespoons soy sauce

Fish sauce

Directions:

1. In a big deep cooking pan, bring the water to its boiling point, then mix in the rice. Cover, decrease the heat to low, and cook until the water is absorbed, approximately twenty minutes.

2. Place the cooked rice in a big mixing container and let cool completely.

3. Put in the ground beef and soy sauce to the rice, mixing meticulously. (I find using my hands works best.)

4. Split the rice-beef mixture into 8 to 12 equivalent portions, depending on the size you prefer, and form them into loose balls. Cover each ball in foil, ensuring to secure them well.

5. Steam the rice balls for twenty-five to thirty minutes or until thoroughly cooked.

6. While the rice is steaming, heat the vegetable oil in a small frying pan. Put in the garlic and the dried chilies and sauté until the garlic is golden. Move the garlic and the chilies to a paper towel to drain.

7. To serve, remove the rice packets from the foil, slightly smash them, and put on serving plates. Pass the garlic-chili mixture, the green onions, and the fish sauce separately to be used as condiments at the table.

Yield: Servings 4–6

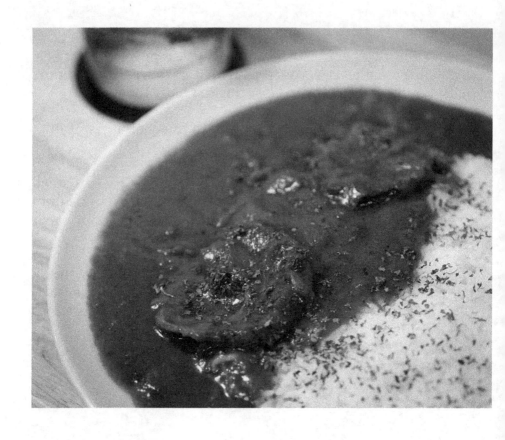

BARBECUED PORK ON RICE

Ingredients:

1 cucumber, thinly cut

1 green onion, trimmed and thinly cut

1 hard-boiled egg, peeled

1 pork tenderloin, trimmed of surplus fat

1 tablespoon sesame seeds, toasted

1 teaspoon Chinese 5-spice powder

1½ cups water

2 tablespoons flour

2 tablespoons rice vinegar

2 tablespoons soy sauce

2 tablespoons sugar

Jasmine rice, cooked in accordance with package directions

Directions:

1. Cut the tenderloin into medallions roughly ¼-inch thick. Put the medallions in a mixing container.

33

2. Mix the sugar, soy sauce, and 5-spice powder in a small container.

3. Pour the soy mixture over pork strips and toss the strips until meticulously coated. Let marinate minimum 30 minutes, but if possible overnight.

4. Preheat your oven to 350 degrees. Put the pork pieces in a single layer on a baking sheet lined using foil. Reserve any remaining marinade.

5. Bake the pork for roughly 1 hour. The pork with be firm and rather dry, but not burned. It will also have a reddish color.

6. Put the reserved marinade in a small deep cooking pan and heat to boiling. Remove the heat and put in the peeled egg, rolling it in the sauce to color it. Take away the egg and set it aside. When sufficiently cool to handle, cut it into thin pieces.

7. Mix the flour and water, and put in it to the marinade. Bring to its boiling point to thicken, then turn off the heat.

8. Put in the vinegar and the sesame seeds. Adjust seasoning by putting in additional sugar and/or soy sauce.

9. To serve, place some Jasmine rice in the middle of each plate. Fan a few pieces of the pork around 1 side of the rice. Fan some cucumber slices and cut hard-boiled egg around the other side.

Ladle some of the sauce over the pork and drizzle with the green onion slices.

Yield: Servings 2–3

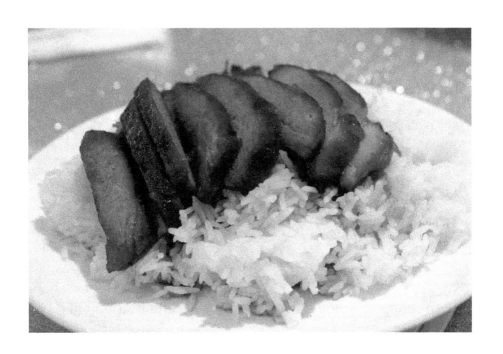

LEMONGRASS PORK

Ingredients:

¼ cup chopped shallots

¼ cup coconut milk

¼ cup minced garlic

¼ cup whiskey

½ cup brown sugar

½ cup chopped lemongrass stalks (inner white portion only)

½ cup dark soy sauce

½ cup fish sauce

1 pound lean pork, cut into bite-sized pieces

1 teaspoon cayenne pepper

3 tablespoons sesame oil

Directions:

1. In a moderate-sized-sized deep cooking pan, mix the brown sugar, fish sauce, soy sauce, lemongrass, whiskey, shallots, and garlic. Over moderate heat, bring to its boiling point and cook until the mixture is reduced to half. Take away the marinade from the heat and let it cool to room temperature. Mix in the coconut milk, sesame oil, and cayenne pepper.

2. Put the pork and the marinade in a big Ziplock bag. Marinate the pork in your fridge for minimum three hours, or overnight.

3. Drain the meat, saving for later the marinade. Thread the meat onto metal skewers (or soaked bamboo skewers), and grill or broil to your preference.

4. Put the reserved marinade in a small deep cooking pan and bring it to its boiling point on moderate to high heat. Lower the heat

 and simmer the marinade for two to three minutes. Use the marinade as a dipping sauce for the pork.

Yield: Servings 2

PORK AND SPINACH CURRY

Ingredients:

½ cup lean pork strips

½ lime

½ pound baby spinach

1 cup coconut milk, divided

1 tablespoon Red Curry Paste (Page 17)

2 cups water

2 tablespoons sugar

3–4 kaffir lime leaves, crumbled

4 tablespoons fish sauce

Rice, cooked in accordance with package directions

Directions:

1. In a moderate-sized-sized deep cooking pan, heat ½ cup of the coconut milk and the curry paste on moderate to low heat, stirring to blend meticulously. Cook for five minutes, stirring continuously, so that the sauce does not burn.

2. Put in the pork cubes, the rest of the coconut milk, and the water. Return the mixture to a simmer and allow to cook for five

minutes. Squeeze the juice of the lime half into the curry. Put in the lime half.

3. Mix in the kaffir lime leaves, fish sauce, and sugar. Continue simmering for five to 10 more minutes or until the pork is thoroughly cooked. Take away the lime half.

4. Put in the baby spinach and cook for a minute.

5. Serve over rice.

Yield: Servings 1–2

THAI-STYLE BEEF WITH BROCCOLI

Ingredients:

½ of a 7–8-ounce package of rice sticks 1 cup broccoli pieces

1 medium shallot, chopped

1 pound lean beef, cut into bite-sized pieces

1 tablespoon preserved soy beans (not necessary)

1 teaspoon chili powder

2 cups water

2 tablespoons brown sugar

2 tablespoons fish sauce

2 tablespoons sweet soy sauce

3 tablespoons vegetable oil

Hot sauce (not necessary)

Lime wedges (not necessary)

Directions:

1. Heat the vegetable oil in a wok on moderate to high heat. Put in the shallot and stir-fry until it starts to become tender. Put in the chili powder and continue to stir-fry until well blended.

2. Put in the brown sugar, fish sauce, soy sauce, and soy beans; stir-fry for half a minute.

3. Put in the beef and continue to stir-fry until the beef is almost done, roughly two minutes.

4. Mix in the water and bring it to its boiling point. Put in the rice sticks, stirring until they start to cook. Lower the heat to moderate, cover, and allow to cook for half a minute. Stir and decrease the heat to moderate-low, cover, and allow to cook for about three minutes.

5. Put in the broccoli pieces, cover, and cook for a minute. Take

 away the wok from the heat and tweak seasoning to taste.

6. Serve with wedges of lime and hot sauce passed separately at the table.

Yield: Servings 2–4

PORK WITH TOMATOES AND STICKY RICE

Ingredients:

½ pound crudely chopped lean pork

½ teaspoon salt

½ teaspoon shrimp paste

1 tablespoon chopped garlic

1 tablespoon fish sauce

1 tablespoon vegetable oil

1 teaspoon brown sugar

2 tablespoons chopped shallot

20 cherry tomatoes, quartered

7 small dried chilies

Sticky rice, cooked in accordance with package directions

Directions:

1. Trim the chilies of their stems and shake out the seeds. Cut them into little pieces, cover them with warm water, and allow them to soak for about twenty minutes to tenderize; drain.

2. Using a food processor or mortar and pestle, grind (or process) the chilies and salt together until a thick paste is

formed. Put in the shrimp paste, shallot, and garlic. Process until well blended; set aside.

3. Heat a wok or heavy-bottomed frying pan using low heat. Put in the vegetable oil and heat for a minute. Put in the chili purée and cook for roughly three minutes or until the color of the paste deepens.

4. Raise the heat to moderate and put in the pork; stir-fry for a

 minute. Put in the tomatoes and carry on cooking for three to four minutes, stirring regularly.

5. Mix in the fish sauce and brown sugar; simmer for a couple of minutes. Adjust seasoning to taste.

6. Serve this beef dish with sticky rice either warm or at room temperature.

Yield: Servings 2

CINNAMON STEWED BEEF

Ingredients:

1 (2-inch) piece of cinnamon stick

1 bay leaf

1 celery stalk, cut

1 clove garlic, smashed

1 pound beef sirloin, trimmed of all fat and slice into 1-inch cubes

1½ quarts water

2 tablespoons sugar

2 tablespoons sweet soy sauce

2 whole star anise

5 sprigs cilantro

5 tablespoons soy sauce

Directions:

1. Put the water in a big soup pot and bring to its boiling point. Decrease the heat to low and put in the rest of the ingredients.
2. Simmer, putting in more water if required, for minimum 2 hours or until the beef is completely soft. If possible, let the stewed beef sit in your fridge overnight.

3. To serve, place noodles or rice on the bottom of 4 soup bowls. Put in pieces of beef and then ladle broth over. Drizzle with chopped cilantro or cut green onions if you prefer. Pass a

vinegar-chili sauce of your choice as a dip for the beef.

Yield: Servings 4

BASIL CHICKEN

Ingredients:

1 big onion, cut into thin slices

1 tablespoon water

1½ cups chopped basil leaves, divided

1½ tablespoons soy sauce

1½ teaspoons sugar

2 tablespoons fish sauce

2 tablespoons vegetable oil

2 whole boneless, skinless chicken breasts, cut into 1-inch cubes

3 cloves garlic, minced

3 Thai chilies, seeded and thinly cut

Directions:

1. In a moderate-sized-sized container, mix the fish sauce, the soy sauce, water, and sugar. Put in the chicken cubes and stir to coat. Let marinate for about ten minutes.

2. In a big frying pan or wok, heat oil on moderate to high heat. Put in the onion and stir-fry for two to three minutes. Put in the chilies and garlic and carry on cooking for another half a minute.

3. Using a slotted spoon, remove the chicken from the marinade and put in it to the frying pan (reserve the marinade.) Stir-fry until almost thoroughly cooked, approximately 3 minutes.
4. Put in the reserved marinade and cook for another half a minute. Take away the frying pan from the heat and mix in 1 cup of the basil.

5. Decorate using the rest of the basil, and serve with rice.

Yield: Servings 4

BRANDIED CHICKEN

Ingredients:

¼ cup vegetable oil

1 (1-inch) piece ginger, cut

1 teaspoon salt

1 whole roasting chicken, washed and trimmed of surplus fat

2 shots brandy

2 tablespoons black soy sauce

6 tablespoons soy sauce

8 cloves garlic, minced

Directions:

1. Fill a pot big enough to hold the whole chicken roughly full of water. Bring the water to its boiling point using high heat. Lower the heat to moderate and cautiously put in the chicken to the pot. Regulate the heat so that the water is just simmering.

2. Poach the whole chicken for twenty minutes to half an hour or until thoroughly cooked. Cautiously remove the chicken from the pot, ensuring to drain the hot water from the cavity of the bird. Position the chicken aside to cool.

3. Take away the skin from the bird and discard. Take away the meat from the chicken and cut it into 1-inch pieces; set aside. (This portion of the recipe can be done 1 or 2 days in advance.)
4. Put in the oil to a big frying pan or wok and heat on medium. Put in the soy sauces, salt, and garlic. Stir-fry until the garlic starts to tenderize, approximately half a minute to one minute.

5. Put in the chicken pieces, stirring to coat. Mix in the brandy and the ginger.

6. Cover the frying pan or wok, decrease the heat to low, and simmer five to ten more minutes.

Yield: Servings 4–6

CHICKEN WITH BLACK PEPPER AND GARLIC

Ingredients:

1 cup fish sauce

1 tablespoon whole black peppercorns

1 teaspoon sugar

2 pounds boneless, skinless chicken breasts, cut into strips

3 tablespoons vegetable oil

5 cloves garlic, cut in half

Directions:

1. Using either a mortar and pestle or a food processor, mix the black peppercorns with the garlic.

2. Put the chicken strips in a big mixing container. Put in the garlic-pepper mixture and the fish sauce, and stir until blended.

3. Cover the container, place in your fridge, and let marinate for twenty minutes to half an hour.

4. Heat the vegetable oil on moderate heat in a wok or frying pan. When it is hot, put in the chicken mixture and stir-fry until thoroughly cooked, approximately 3 to five minutes.

5. Mix in the sugar. Put in additional sugar or fish sauce to taste.

Yield: Servings 4–6

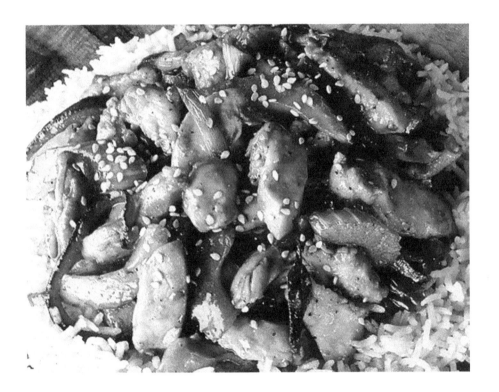

CHILI-FRIED CHICKEN

Ingredients:

½ teaspoon ground coriander

½ teaspoon white pepper

1½ teaspoons salt, divided

2 small onions, thinly cut

2 tablespoons vegetable oil

3 pounds chicken pieces, washed and patted dry

3 tablespoons Tamarind Concentrate (Page 20)

8 big red chilies, seeded and chopped

Pinch of turmeric

Vegetable oil for deep-frying

Directions:

1. In a small container mix the tamarind, turmeric, coriander, 1 teaspoon of the salt, and the pepper.

2. Put the chicken pieces in a big Ziplock bag. Pour the tamarind mixture over the chicken, seal the bag, and marinate minimum 2 hours or overnight in your fridge.

3. In a small sauté pan, heat 2 tablespoons of vegetable oil on moderate heat. Put in the red chilies, onions, and the rest of the salt; sauté for five minutes. Set aside to cool slightly.

4. Move the chili mixture to a food processor and pulse for a short period of time to make a coarse sauce.

5. Drain the chicken and discard the marinade. Deep-fry the chicken pieces in hot oil until the skin is golden and the bones are crunchy. Take away the cooked chicken to paper towels to drain.

6. Put the cooked chicken in a big mixing container. Pour the chili sauce over the chicken and toss until each piece is uniformly coated.

Yield: Servings 4–6

FRAGRANT ROAST CHICKEN

Ingredients:

For the marinade:

½ cup fish sauce

½ cup sweet dark soy sauce

1 tablespoon freshly ground black pepper

2 tablespoons crushed garlic

2 tablespoons freshly grated gingerroot

For the stuffing:

½ cup chopped cilantro

½ cup chopped mushrooms

½ cup cut bruised lemongrass stalks

½ cup fresh grated galangal

½ cup freshly grated ginger

1 roasting chicken, cleaned and patted dry

Directions:

1. Mix all of the marinade ingredients in a plastic bag big enough to hold the whole chicken. Put in the chicken, ensuring to coat the whole bird with the marinade. Put the chicken in your fridge and leave overnight.

2. Take away the chicken from the plastic bag, saving for later the marinade.

3. Put all of the stuffing ingredients in a big mixing container. Mix in the reserved marinade.

4. Fill the bird's cavity and place it breast side up in a roasting pan. Put the roasting pan in a preheated 400 degree oven and roast for 50 to 60 minutes, or until the juices run clear.

Yield: Servings 2–4

GINGER CHICKEN

Ingredients:

1 cup cut domestic mushrooms

1 tablespoon chopped garlic

1 whole boneless, skinless chicken breast, cut into bite-sized pieces

2 tablespoons dark soy sauce

2 tablespoons fish sauce

2 tablespoons oyster sauce

2–3 habanero or bird's eye chilis

3 green onions, trimmed and slice into 1-inch pieces

3 tablespoons chopped onion

3 tablespoons grated ginger

3 tablespoons vegetable oil

Cilantro

Jasmine rice, cooked in accordance with package directions
Pinch of sugar

Directions:

1. In a small container mix the fish, soy, and oyster sauces; set aside.

2. Heat the oil in a big wok until super hot. Put in the garlic and chicken, and stir-fry just until the chicken starts to change color.

3. Put in the reserved sauce and cook until it starts to simmer while stirring continuously.

4. Put in the mushrooms, ginger, sugar, onion, and chilies; simmer until the chicken is thoroughly cooked, approximately eight minutes.

5. To serve, ladle the chicken over Jasmine rice and top with green onion and cilantro.

Yield: Servings 2

JUNGLE CHICKEN

Ingredients:

½ cup coconut milk

1 stalk lemongrass, inner portion roughly chopped

1 whole boneless, skinless chicken breast, cut into fine strips 10–fifteen basil leaves

 2 (2-inch-long, ½-inch wide) strips of lime peel

2 tablespoons vegetable oil

2–4 serrano chilies, stems and seeds removed 2–4 tablespoons fish sauce

Directions:

1. Put the chilies, lemongrass, and lime peel into a food processor and pulse until ground.

2. Heat the oil on moderate to high heat in a wok or big frying pan. Put in the chili mixture and sauté for one to two minutes.

3. Mix in the coconut milk and cook for a couple of minutes.

4. Put in the chicken and cook until the chicken is thoroughly cooked, approximately five minutes.

5. Decrease the heat to low and put in the fish sauce and basil leaves to taste.

6. Serve with sufficient Jasmine rice.

Yield: Servings 2–3

LEMONGRASS CHICKEN SKEWERS

Ingredients:

12 big cubes chicken breast meat, a little over 1 ounce each

2 tablespoons vegetable oil, divided

2 teaspoons fish sauce

5 stalks lemongrass, trimmed

Black pepper

Juice of 1 lime

Pinch of dried red pepper flakes

Pinch of sugar

Sea salt to taste

Directions:

1. Remove 2 inches from the thick end of each stalk of lemongrass; set aside. Bruise 4 of the lemongrass stalks using the back of a knife. Take away the tough outer layer of the fifth stalk, exposing the soft core; mince.

2. Skewer 3 cubes of chicken on each lemongrass stalk. Drizzle the skewers with the minced lemongrass and black pepper, and sprinkle with 1 tablespoon of oil. Cover using plastic wrap and place in your fridge for twelve to one day.

3. Chop all of the reserved lemongrass stalk ends. Put in a small deep cooking pan and cover with water. Bring to its boiling point, cover, and let reduce until roughly 2 tablespoons of liquid is left; strain. Return the liquid to the deep cooking pan and further reduce to 1 tablespoon.

4. Mix the lemongrass liquid with the red pepper flakes, lime juice, fish sauce, sugar, and remaining tablespoon of oil; set aside.
5. Prepare a grill to high heat. Grill the chicken skewers for roughly two to three minutes per side, or until done to your preference.

6. To serve, spoon a little of the lemongrass sauce over the top of each skewer and drizzle with sea salt.

Yield: Servings 4

RED CHILI CHICKEN

Ingredients:

1 tablespoon vegetable oil

½ cup coconut milk

1 whole boneless, skinless chicken breast, cut into bite-sized pieces

2 kaffir lime leaves or 2 (2-inch-long, ½–inch wide) pieces of lime zest

1 tablespoon basil leaves

2 tablespoons fish sauce

1 tablespoon brown sugar

4 ounces Thai eggplant (green peas can be substituted)

1–3 tablespoons Red Curry Paste (Page 17)

Directions:

1. In a big frying pan or wok, heat the oil on moderate to high heat. Mix in the curry paste and cook until aromatic, approximately one minute.

2. Lower the heat to moderate-low and put in the coconut milk. Stirring continuously, cook until a thin film of oil develops on the surface.

3. Put in all of the rest of the ingredients except the eggplant. Bring to its boiling point, reduce heat, and simmer until the chicken starts to turn opaque, approximately five minutes.

4. Put in the eggplant and carry on cooking until the chicken is done to your preference, approximately 3 minutes more.

Yield: Servings 2

THAI ROAST CHICKEN

Ingredients:

1 clove garlic, minced

1 medium onion, chopped

1 tablespoon fish sauce

1 teaspoon (or to taste) dried red pepper flakes

1 whole roasting chicken

2 stalks lemongrass, thinly cut (soft inner core only)

Salt and pepper to taste

Vegetable oil

Directions:

1. To prepare the marinade, put the lemongrass, onion, garlic, red pepper, and fish sauce in a food processor. Process until a thick

 paste is formed. Place in your fridge for minimum 30 minutes, overnight if possible.

2. Spread the marinade throughout the chicken cavity and then drizzle the cavity with salt and pepper. Rub the outside of the bird with a small amount of vegetable oil (or butter if you prefer) and sprinkle with salt and pepper. Put the bird in a roasting pan, and cover it using plastic wrap. Place in your fridge for a few

64

hours to marinate, if possible. Take away the chicken from the fridge roughly thirty minutes before roasting.

3. Preheat your oven to 500 degrees. Take away the plastic wrap and put the bird in your oven, legs first, and roast for 50 to 60 minutes or until the juices run clear.

Yield: Servings 2–4

SWEET-AND-SOUR CHICKEN

Ingredients:

1 (1-inch) piece of ginger, peeled and minced

1 green and 1 red bell pepper, seeded and slice into 1-inch pieces

1 pound boneless, skinless chicken breasts, cut into 1-inch cubes

1 small onion, thinly cut

1 tablespoon vegetable oil

1–2 tablespoons prepared chili sauce

2 cloves garlic, minced

2 tablespoons soy sauce

4–6 tablespoons prepared Plum Sauce

8 ounces canned pineapple pieces, drained

Jasmine rice, cooked in accordance with package directions

Directions:

1. In a small container, mix the soy sauce, garlic, ginger, and chili sauce. Put in the chicken pieces, stirring to coat. Set aside to

marinate for minimum twenty minutes.

2. Heat the oil in a wok or big frying pan on moderate heat. Put in the onion and sauté until translucent, approximately 3 minutes.

3. Put in the chicken mixture and carry on cooking for another three to five minutes.

4. Put in the bell peppers, the pineapple, and plum sauce. Cook for another five minutes or until the chicken is thoroughly cooked.

5. Serve over lots of fluffy Jasmine rice.

Yield: Servings 4

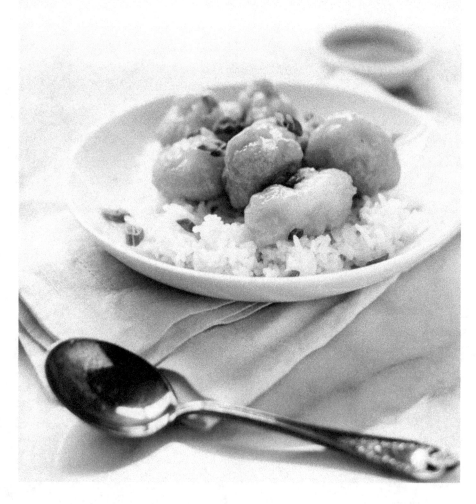

TAMARIND STIR-FRIED CHICKEN WITH MUSHROOMS

Ingredients:

2 tablespoons vegetable oil

Salt and freshly ground black pepper

1 teaspoon sugar

4 ounces domestic mushrooms, cut

½ cup cut onions

1 clove garlic, minced

2 tablespoons <u>Tamarind Concentrate</u>

2 tablespoons water

1 cup bean sprouts

1 small jalapeño, seeded and minced

¼ cup chopped basil

1–2 whole boneless, skinless chicken breasts, cut into bite-sized cubes

Directions:

1. Heat the vegetable oil in a big sauté pan or wok using high heat. Flavour the chicken with the salt, pepper, and sugar.

2. Put in the chicken to the pan and stir-fry for a couple of minutes.

 Put in the mushrooms, onions, and garlic; carry on cooking for another two to three minutes. Put in the tamarind and water; stir.

3. Put in the rest of the ingredients. Adjust seasonings to taste before you serve.

Yield: Servings 1–2

THAI CASHEW CHICKEN

Ingredients:

3 tablespoons vegetable oil

1 big whole boneless, skinless chicken breast, cut into fine strips

4 green onions, trimmed and slice into 1-inch lengths

1 small onion, thinly cut

¼ cup chicken broth

1 tablespoon oyster sauce

1 tablespoon fish sauce

2 tablespoons sugar

¾ cup whole cashews

2–3 teaspoons Chili Tamarind Paste

5–10 dried Thai chilies

5–10 cloves garlic, mashed

Directions:

1. In a wok or big frying pan, heat the oil on moderate to high heat until hot.

2. Put in the chilies and stir-fry for a short period of time until they darken in color. Move the chilies to a paper towel to drain; set aside.

3. Put in the garlic to the wok and stir-fry until just starting to turn golden.

4. Increase the heat to high and put in the chicken. Cook while stirring continuously, for roughly one minute.

5. Put in the green onions and onion slices and cook for half a minute.

6. Put in the Chili Tamarind Paste, broth, oyster sauce, fish sauce, and sugar. Continue to stir-fry for 30 more seconds.

7. Put in the reserved chilies and the cashews; stir-fry for 1 more minute or until the chicken is thoroughly cooked and the onions are soft.

Yield: Servings 2–4

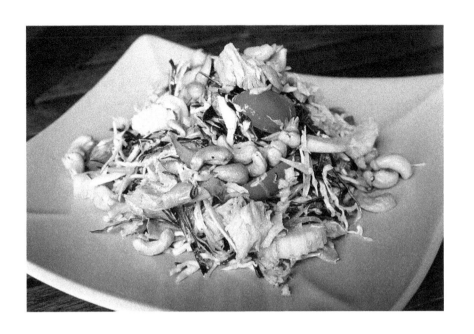

THAI GLAZED CHICKEN

Ingredients:

1 tablespoon fish sauce

1 tablespoon minced cilantro

1 teaspoon chopped ginger

1 teaspoon salt

1 teaspoon white pepper

1 whole chicken, cut in half (ask your butcher to do this for you)

2 tablespoons coconut milk

2 tablespoons rice wine

2 tablespoons soy sauce

4 cloves garlic, chopped

Directions:

1. Wash the chicken under cold water, then pat dry. Trim off any surplus fat or skin. Put the chicken halves in big Ziplock bags.
2. Mix the rest of the ingredients together in a small container until well blended.

3. Pour the marinade into the Ziplock bags, seal closed, and turn until the chicken is uniformly coated with the marinade. Allow

the chicken to marinate for thirty minutes to an hour in your fridge.

4. Preheat your oven to 350 degrees.

5. Take away the chicken from the bags and put them breast side up in a roasting pan big enough to hold them easily. (Discard the rest of the marinade.)

6. Roast the chicken for about forty-five minutes.

7. Turn on the broiler and broil for roughly ten minutes or until done.

Yield: Servings 2–4

THAI-STYLE GREEN CURRY CHICKEN

Ingredients:

¼ cup (or to taste) chopped cilantro leaves ¼ cup Green Curry Paste ¼ cup vegetable oil

2 cups coconut milk

3 tablespoons fish sauce

3 whole boneless, skinless chicken breasts, cut into bite-sized pieces

Steamed white rice

Directions:

1. Heat 2 tablespoons of vegetable oil in a big sauté pan or wok on moderate heat. Put in the chicken and sauté until mildly browned on all sizes. Take away the chicken and save for later.

2. Put in the remaining vegetable oil to the sauté pan. Mix in the curry paste and cook for two to three minutes. Put in the coconut milk and carry on cooking for five minutes. Put in the reserved chicken and fish sauce. Decrease the heat and simmer until chicken is soft, fifteen to twenty minutes. Mix in the cilantro.

3. Serve with steamed white rice.

Yield: Servings 4–6

SKEWERED THAI PORK

Ingredients:

1 pound pork, thinly cut into lengthy strips

1 tablespoon coconut milk

1 tablespoon fish sauce

1 teaspoon salt

2 tablespoons sugar

20–30 bamboo skewers, soaked in water for an hour 3 cloves garlic, minced

Directions:

1. In a moderate-sized-sized container, mix the sugar, salt, garlic, fish sauce, and coconut milk.

2. Toss the pork strips in the mixture to coat completely. Cover the container and marinate for minimum 30 minutes, but if possible overnight in your fridge.

3. Thread the pork strips onto the bamboo skewers.

4. Grill the skewers for approximately 3 to five minutes per side.

5. Serve with your favorite sauce or as is.

Yield: Servings 2–3

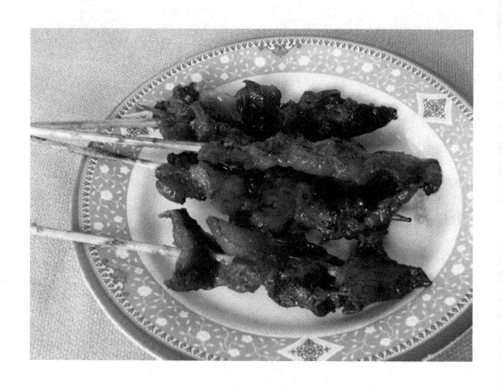

SPICY GROUND PORK IN BASIL LEAVES

Ingredients:

¼ tablespoon (or to taste) ground dried chili pepper

½ pound ground pork

1 shallot, thinly cut

1 tablespoon toasted rice powder (available in Asian specialty stores)

3 tablespoons fish sauce

5 sprigs cilantro, chopped

Juice of 1–2 limes

Lettuce and/or big basil leaves

Directions:

1. Squeeze the juice of half of a lime over the ground pork and let marinate for a few minutes.

2. Heat a big frying pan on high. Put in a couple of tablespoons of water and then instantly put in the pork; stir-fry until the pork is thoroughly cooked. (It is okay if the pork sticks at first — it will ultimately loosen.)

3. Pour off any fat that has collected in the pan and then put the pork in a big mixing container. Put in the remaining lime juice

(to taste), fish sauce, shallot, ground chili pepper, cilantro, and toasted rice; stir until blended meticulously.

4. To serve, put the mixture in a serving container and let guests use the lettuce and basil leaves to scoop out the mixture.

Yield: Servings 4

SPICY SCALLOPS

Ingredients:

1 (½-inch) piece of ginger, peeled and minced

1 clove garlic, minced

1 jalapeño, seeded and minced

1 teaspoon vegetable oil

2 tablespoons soy sauce

2 tablespoons water

8 big scallops, cleaned

teaspoon ground coriander

Directions:

1. In a pan big enough to hold all of the scallops, heat the oil on moderate heat. Put in the garlic, jalapeño, and ginger, and stir-fry for approximately one minute.

2. Put in the coriander, soy sauce, and water, stirring to blend; simmer for two to three minutes. Strain the liquid through a fine-mesh sieve. Allow the pan to cool slightly.

3. Put in the scallops to the pan and spoon the reserved liquid over the top of them. Return the pan to the stove, increasing the heat to moderate-high. Cover the pan and let the scallops steam

for approximately two to three minutes, or until done to your preference. Serve instantly.

Yield: Servings 4

PORK TOAST TRIANGLES

Ingredients:

¼ pound of big shrimp, peeled and deveined 1 egg

1 pound ground pork (the leaner the better)

1 tablespoon chopped cilantro

1 tablespoon dried shrimp

1 tablespoon fish sauce

2 cloves garlic, peeled

6 slices day-old bread, crusts trimmed off Vegetable oil for frying

Directions:

1. Fill a moderate-sized deep cooking pan with water and bring it to its boiling point. Reduce the heat, put in the shrimp, and simmer until the shrimp are opaque. Drain the shrimp and let cool completely. Coarsely cut and save for later.

2. Put the dried shrimp, cilantro, and the garlic in a food processor

and pulse until a smooth paste is formed. Put in the reserved shrimp and ground pork; process once more. Put in the egg and fish sauce and process one more time.

3. Spread the mixture uniformly over each slice of bread. Chop the bread into 4 equal slices, either from corner to corner forming triangles or from top to bottom forming squares.

4. Put in roughly ½ inch of vegetable oil to a big frying pan. Bring the oil to roughly 375 degrees on moderate to high heat. Put 4 to 5 toasts in the oil, filling side down. Ensure that the toasts are not crowded in the oil or they will not brown uniformly. After the filling side is well browned, use a slotted spoon or metal strainer to flip the toasts. Watch the toasts cautiously, as the bottoms will brown swiftly. Take away the toasts to a stack of paper towels to drain. Cautiously pat the tops of the toasts using paper towels to remove any oil.

5. Serve the toasts with sweet-and-sour or plum sauce.

Yield: 24 pieces

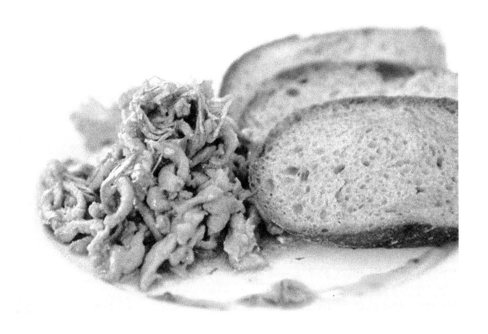

PORK, CARROT, AND CELERY SPRING ROLLS

Ingredients:

¼ cup fish sauce

¼ teaspoon white pepper

1 cup bean sprouts

1 cup minced or ground pork

1 teaspoon minced garlic

2 cups chopped celery

2 cups grated carrots

2 egg yolks, beaten

2 tablespoons sugar

2 tablespoons vegetable oil

20 spring roll wrappers

Vegetable oil for deep frying

Directions:

1. In a big frying pan, heat the 2 tablespoons of vegetable oil over moderatehigh heat. Put in the garlic and pork, and sauté until the pork is thoroughly cooked.

2. Put in the carrots, celery, fish sauce, sugar, and white pepper. Increase heat to high and cook for a minute.

3. Drain any liquid from the pan and allow the mixture to cool completely, then mix in the bean sprouts.

4. On a clean, dry work surface, put the egg roll wrapper with an end pointing toward you, making a diamond. Put roughly 2 tablespoons of the filling on the lower portion of the wrapper. Fold up the corner nearest you and roll once, then fold in the sides. Brush the rest of the point with the egg yolk and finish rolling to secure. Repeat with the rest of the wrappers and filling.
5. Heat 2 to 3 inches of oil to 350 degrees. Deep-fry the spring rolls until a golden-brown colour is achieved; remove instantly to drain using paper towels.

6. Serve with sweet-and-sour sauce.

Yield: 20 rolls

THAI CHICKEN

1 recipe Peanut Dipping Sauce

1 recipe Thai Marinade

3 whole boneless, skinless chicken breasts, cut into lengthy strips about ½-inch wide

Directions:

1. Thread the chicken strips onto presoaked bamboo skewers or onto metal skewers. Put the skewers in a flat pan and cover with

 marinade. Marinate the chicken in your fridge overnight.

2. Cook the skewers on the grill or under the broiler, coating and turning them until they are thoroughly cooked, approximately six to eight minutes.
3. Serve with the peanut sauce for dipping.

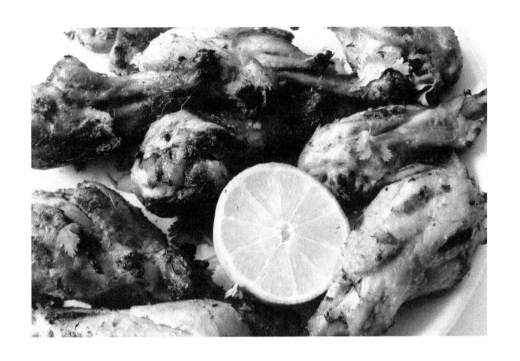

THAI SHRIMP

1 recipe Peanut Dipping Sauce

1 recipe Thai Marinade

24 big shrimp, shelled and deveined

Directions:

1. Thread the shrimp onto presoaked bamboo skewers or onto metal skewers (about 3 shrimp per skewer). Put the skewers in a flat pan and cover with marinade. Marinate the shrimp for minimum fifteen minutes, but no longer than an hour.

2. Cook the skewers on the grill or under the broiler, coating and turning them frequently until just opaque, approximately three to four minutes.

3. Serve with the peanut sauce for dipping.

Yield: 4–6 chicken skewers or 6–8 shrimp or beef skewers

1 recipe Thai Marinade

1 recipe Peanut Dipping Sauce

1-1½ pounds sirloin steak, fat and sinew removed, cut into ½-inch-wide strips

Directions:

1. Thread the beef strips onto presoaked bamboo skewers or onto metal skewers. Put the skewers in a flat pan and cover with marinade. Marinate the beef in your fridge overnight.

2. Cook the skewers on the grill or under the broiler, coating and turning them frequently until done to your preference, approximately six to eight minutes for medium.

3. Serve with the peanut sauce for dipping.

THAI CHICKEN NOODLE SOUP

Ingredients:

½ cup chopped onion

1 carrot, peeled and julienned

1 cup chopped cilantro

1 moderate-sized sweet red pepper, seeded and julienned

2 cups chicken broth

2 star anise

2 tablespoons chopped ginger

2 tablespoons fish sauce

2 tablespoons vegetable oil

2 whole boneless, skinless chicken breasts, cut into lengthy strips

3 cloves garlic, minced

3 ounces snow peas, trimmed

4 ounces, cellophane noodles, soaked in boiling water for five minutes and drained

5 cups water, divided

Lemon or lime wedges

Peanuts, crudely chopped

Directions:

1. In a big deep cooking pan, heat the oil on high. Put in the onion and sauté until translucent. Put in the ginger, garlic, and cilantro, and sauté for 1 more minute. Mix in the broth and 2 cups of the water. Put in the star anise. Bring to its boiling point, reduce heat, and cover; simmer for twenty minutes to half an hour.

2. In another deep cooking pan, bring the rest of the water to its boiling point. Put in the vegetables and blanch for a minute or until soft-crisp. Drain and run very cold water over the

 vegetables to stop the cooking process; set aside.

3. Strain the broth into a clean soup pot and bring to its boiling point. Put in the chicken strips and reduce heat. Poach the chicken using low heat until opaque, roughly ten minutes. Put in the cellophane noodles and reserved vegetables, and carry on simmering for two more minutes. Season to taste with fish sauce.

4. To serve, ladle the soup into warm bowls. Drizzle with peanuts and decorate with lime wedge.

Yield: Servings 4 to 6

CHICKEN SOUP WITH LEMONGRASS

Ingredients:

¾ pound boneless, skinless chicken breast, trimmed and slice into bite-sized pieces

1 (14-ounce) can unsweetened coconut milk

1 (1-inch) piece ginger, cut into 6 pieces

1 clove garlic, minced

1 medium onion, minced

1 stalk lemongrass, trimmed, bruised, and slice into 2 to 3 pieces

1 tablespoon vegetable oil

2 cups wild or domestic mushrooms, cut into bite-sized pieces (if required)

2 tablespoons fish sauce

2 teaspoons prepared <u>Red Curry Paste</u> or curry powder

3 lime leaves (fresh or dried)

4 cups chicken broth

Juice of 2 limes

Salt and pepper to taste

Directions:

1. In a moderate-sized-sized deep cooking pan, mix the oil, onion,

and garlic. Cook on moderate heat for a minute. Put in the lemongrass, curry paste, ginger, and lime leaves.

2. Cook while stirring, for about three minutes, then put in the broth. Bring to its boiling point, decrease the heat to moderate, and carry on cooking for ten more minutes.

3. Put in the coconut milk, the chicken pieces, and the mushrooms. Continue to cook for five minutes or until the chicken is done.
4. Mix in the lime juice and fish sauce. Sprinkle salt and pepper to taste.

5. Take away the lemongrass, lime leaves, and ginger pieces before you serve.

Yield: Servings 4–6

THAI-SPICED BEEF SOUP WITH RICE NOODLES

Ingredients:

¼ cup fish sauce

¾ cup leftover beef roast, chopped or shredded 1 (2–inch) cinnamon stick

1 stalk lemongrass, tough outer leaves removed, inner core crushed and minced

1 tablespoon prepared chiligarlic sauce

1 whole star anise, crushed

2 (¼–inch) pieces peeled gingerroot

2½ tablespoons lime juice

3–4 teaspoons (or to taste) salt

8 cups beef broth

8 ounces rice noodles, soaked in hot water for approximately ten minutes, strained and washed in cold water Freshly ground black pepper to taste

Directions:

1. In a moderate-sized-sized deep cooking pan, simmer the beef broth, star anise, cinnamon stick, and ginger using low heat for thirty to forty minutes.

2. Strain the stock and return to the deep cooking pan.

3. Put in the noodles, lemongrass, shredded beef, fish sauce, chili sauce, and garlic. Bring the soup to its boiling point on moderate heat. Decrease the heat and simmer for five minutes. Mix in the lime juice, salt, and pepper.

Yield: Servings 4–6

TOM KA KAI

Ingredients:

1 (1-inch) piece ginger, cut thinly

1 (2-inch) piece of lemongrass, bruised

1 boneless, skinless chicken breast, cut into bite-sized pieces

1 teaspoon cut kaffir lime leaves

2 cups chicken broth

2 tablespoons lime juice

2–4 Thai chilies (to taste), slightly crushed 4 tablespoons fish sauce 5 ounces coconut milk

Directions:

1. In a moderate-sized-sized soup pot, heat the broth on medium. Put in the lime leaves, lemongrass, ginger, fish sauce, and lime juice.

2. Bring the mixture to its boiling point, put in the chicken and coconut milk, and bring to its boiling point once more.

3. Reduce the heat, put in the chilies, and cover; allow to simmer until the chicken is thoroughly cooked, approximately 3 to five minutes.

4. Take away the chilies and the lemongrass stalk using a slotted spoon before you serve.
Yield: Servings 4–6

CHICKEN BREAST WITH PEANUT SAUCE AND NOODLES

Ingredients:

¼ cup chicken stock

¼ cup lime juice

¼cup half-and-half

1 cup crispy peanut butter

1 pound Chinese egg noodles (mein)

1 pound snow peas, trimmed and blanched

1 tablespoon peanut oil

1 tablespoon sesame oil

1½ cups coconut milk

2 tablespoons fish sauce

2 teaspoons brown sugar

3 whole boneless, skinless chicken breasts, halved and poached

4 cloves garlic, minced

6–8 green onions, trimmed and thinly cut Salt and pepper to taste

Directions:

1. Mix the peanut butter, coconut milk, fish sauce, lime juice, brown sugar, garlic, salt, and pepper in a small deep cooking pan using low heat. Cook until the desired smoothness is achieved and thick, stirring regularly.

2. Move to a blender and purée.

3. Put in the chicken stock and half-and-half, and blend; set aside.

4. Bring a big pot of water to its boiling point. Put in the noodles and cook until firm to the bite. Drain, wash under cold water, and drain once more.

5. Toss the noodles with the peanut and sesame oils.

6. To serve, place some pasta in the center of each serving plate. Ladle some of the peanut sauce over the pasta. Slice each chicken breast on the diagonal. Move 1 cut breast to the top of each portion of noodles. Ladle some additional peanut sauce over the chicken. Surround the noodles with the snow peas. Decorate using the cut green onions.

Yield: Servings 6

NOODLES WITH CHICKEN AND VEGETABLES

Ingredients:

Noodles:

1 tablespoon sweet black soy sauce

2 tablespoons vegetable oil

8 ounces rice stick noodles

Chicken and vegetables:

¼ cup chicken broth

¼– cup cut green onions

¼ pound broccoli, chopped

½ teaspoon Tabasco

1 big whole boneless, skinless chicken breast, cut into bite-sized strips

1 cup bean sprouts

1 small onion, finely cut

1 small red bell pepper, seeded and slice into strips

1 tablespoon cornstarch mixed with

1 tablespoon water

1¼ cups cut Japanese eggplant

2 tablespoons fish sauce

2 tablespoons vegetable oil

2 tablespoons <u>Yellow Bean Sauce (Page 24)</u>

3 tablespoons brown sugar

4 cloves garlic, chopped

Yield: Servings 2–4

THAI NOODLES

1. Soak the noodles in warm water for fifteen minutes or until soft; drain.

2. Put a wok on moderate to high heat and put in the vegetable oil. Once the oil is hot, put in the noodles and stir-fry vigorously until they are thoroughly heated, approximately 45 seconds to one minute.

3. Put in the soy sauce and continue to stir-fry for 1 more minute.

4. Put the noodles on a serving platter, covered in foil, in a warm oven until ready to serve.

THAI CHICKEN AND VEGETABLES:

1. Put a wok on moderate to high heat and put in the vegetable oil. Once the oil is hot, put in the garlic and stir-fry for a short period of time to release its aroma.

2. Put in the chicken and cook until it begins to become opaque.

3. Put in the broccoli and stir-fry for half a minute.

4. Put in the onion and eggplant and stir-fry for a couple of minutes.

5. Put in the Tabasco, fish sauce, yellow bean sauce, and sugar. Stir-fry for a minute.

6. Put in the broth, cornstarch mixture, bean sprouts, green onions, and red bell pepper; cook until vegetables are soft-crisp.

7. To serve, ladle the chicken and vegetable mixture over the reserved noodles.

SPICY EGG NOODLES WITH SLICED PORK

Ingredients:

½ teaspoon vegetable oil

1 cup bean sprouts

1 package fresh angel hair pasta

1 small Barbecued Pork

1 small cabbage, shredded

2 scallions, trimmed and thinly cut

2 tablespoons fish sauce

2 tablespoons sugar

2 teaspoons chopped cilantro

2 teaspoons ground dried red chili pepper (or to taste)

4 tablespoons minced garlic

4–6 tablespoons rice vinegar

Freshly ground black pepper to taste

Tenderloin, thinly cut

Directions:

1. Bring a big pot of water to its boiling point using high heat. Put in the cabbage and blanch about half a minute. Using a slotted spoon, remove the cabbage from the boiling water; set aside.

2. Allow the water return to boiling. Put in the bean sprouts and blanch for ten seconds. Using a slotted spoon, remove the sprouts from the water; set aside.

3. Return the water to boiling. Put in the fresh angel hair pasta and cook in accordance with package directions. Drain the pasta and place it in a big mixing container.

4. In a small sauté pan, heat the vegetable oil on moderate heat. Put in the garlic and sauté until golden. Turn off the heat. Mix in the fish sauce, sugar, rice vinegar, and dried chili pepper.

5. Pour the sauce over the pasta and toss to coat.

6. To serve, split the cabbage and the bean sprouts into 2 to 4 portions and place in the middle of serving plates. Split the noodles into 2 to 4 portions and place over the cabbage and sprouts. Split the pork slices over the noodles. Grind black pepper to taste over the noodles and top with the cut scallions and chopped cilantro.

Yield: Servings 2 as a main course or 4 as an appetizer.

THAI NOODLES WITH CHICKEN AND PORK

Ingredients:

For the sauce:

¼ teaspoon white pepper

½ cup peanut butter

½ cup soy sauce

1 teaspoon hot chili oil

1 teaspoon minced garlic

3 tablespoons honey

3 tablespoons sesame oil

For the noodles:

½ pound boneless pork tenderloin, cut into fine strips

½ pound boneless, skinless chicken breast, cut thin

½ teaspoon minced garlic

1 big yellow onion, diced

1 pound dry flat Asian noodles

1 tablespoon vegetable oil

1 teaspoon sesame oil

6 ounces salad shrimp

6–8 green onions, trimmed, white portions cut, green portions julienned

Directions:

1. Put all of the sauce ingredients in a blender and pulse until smooth; set aside.

2. Bring a big pot of water to boil using high heat. Prepare the noodles in accordance with package directions, drain, and mix in the sauce mixture, saving for later ¼ cup; set aside.

3. Heat the oils in a big sautée pan using high heat. Put in the garlic and sautée for a short period of time.

4. Put in the chicken, pork, and onion, and sauté for five to six minutes or until the meats are thoroughly cooked.

5. Put in the white portion of the green onion and the shrimp and sautée for two more minutes.

6. Put in the green parts of the onions and the rest of the sauce, stirring until everything is thoroughly coated.

7. To serve, put the noodles on a big platter and top with the meat sautée. Pass additional hot chili oil separately.

Yield: Servings 4–6

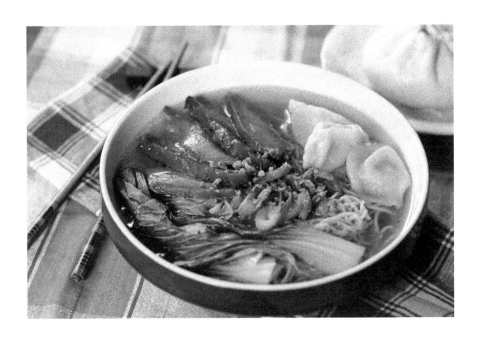

CPSIA information can be obtained
at www.ICGtesting.com
Printed in the USA
BVHW090034280421
605944BV00005B/932